Blood Sugar

BELONGS TO:

_____

EMERGENCY CONTACTS:

_____

_____

_____

ESSENTIAL CONTACTS:

_____

_____

_____

OTHER INFO:

_____

_____

_____

Week Commencing _____   Feeling _____ / 10

	Breakfast		Lunch		Dinner		Supper
	BEFORE	AFTER	BEFORE	AFTER	BEFORE	AFTER	BEFORE
M							
NOTES							
	BEFORE	AFTER	BEFORE	AFTER	BEFORE	AFTER	BEFORE
T							
NOTES							
	BEFORE	AFTER	BEFORE	AFTER	BEFORE	AFTER	BEFORE
W							
NOTES							
	BEFORE	AFTER	BEFORE	AFTER	BEFORE	AFTER	BEFORE
T							
NOTES							
	BEFORE	AFTER	BEFORE	AFTER	BEFORE	AFTER	BEFORE
F							
NOTES							
	BEFORE	AFTER	BEFORE	AFTER	BEFORE	AFTER	BEFORE
S							
NOTES							
	BEFORE	AFTER	BEFORE	AFTER	BEFORE	AFTER	BEFORE
S							
NOTES							

Week Commencing _____   Feeling _____ / 10

	Breakfast		Lunch		Dinner		Supper
	BEFORE	AFTER	BEFORE	AFTER	BEFORE	AFTER	BEFORE
M							
NOTES							
	BEFORE	AFTER	BEFORE	AFTER	BEFORE	AFTER	BEFORE
T							
NOTES							
	BEFORE	AFTER	BEFORE	AFTER	BEFORE	AFTER	BEFORE
W							
NOTES							
	BEFORE	AFTER	BEFORE	AFTER	BEFORE	AFTER	BEFORE
T							
NOTES							
	BEFORE	AFTER	BEFORE	AFTER	BEFORE	AFTER	BEFORE
F							
NOTES							
	BEFORE	AFTER	BEFORE	AFTER	BEFORE	AFTER	BEFORE
S							
NOTES							
	BEFORE	AFTER	BEFORE	AFTER	BEFORE	AFTER	BEFORE
S							
NOTES							

Week Commencing _____   Feeling _____ / 10

	Breakfast		Lunch		Dinner		Supper
	BEFORE	AFTER	BEFORE	AFTER	BEFORE	AFTER	BEFORE
M							
NOTES							
T							
NOTES							
W							
NOTES							
T							
NOTES							
F							
NOTES							
S							
NOTES							
S							
NOTES							

Week Commencing _____   Feeling ___ / 10

	Breakfast		Lunch		Dinner		Supper
	BEFORE	AFTER	BEFORE	AFTER	BEFORE	AFTER	BEFORE
M							
NOTES							
T							
NOTES							
W							
NOTES							
T							
NOTES							
F							
NOTES							
S							
NOTES							
S							
NOTES							

Week Commencing _____   Feeling ____ / 10

	Breakfast		Lunch		Dinner		Supper
	BEFORE	AFTER	BEFORE	AFTER	BEFORE	AFTER	BEFORE
M NOTES							
T NOTES							
W NOTES							
T NOTES							
F NOTES							
S NOTES							
S NOTES							

Week Commencing _____   Feeling ____ / 10

	Breakfast		Lunch		Dinner		Supper
	BEFORE	AFTER	BEFORE	AFTER	BEFORE	AFTER	BEFORE
M							
NOTES							
T	BEFORE	AFTER	BEFORE	AFTER	BEFORE	AFTER	BEFORE
NOTES							
W	BEFORE	AFTER	BEFORE	AFTER	BEFORE	AFTER	BEFORE
NOTES							
T	BEFORE	AFTER	BEFORE	AFTER	BEFORE	AFTER	BEFORE
NOTES							
F	BEFORE	AFTER	BEFORE	AFTER	BEFORE	AFTER	BEFORE
NOTES							
S	BEFORE	AFTER	BEFORE	AFTER	BEFORE	AFTER	BEFORE
NOTES							
S	BEFORE	AFTER	BEFORE	AFTER	BEFORE	AFTER	BEFORE
NOTES							

Week Commencing _____   Feeling ___ / 10

	Breakfast		Lunch		Dinner		Supper
	BEFORE	AFTER	BEFORE	AFTER	BEFORE	AFTER	BEFORE
M NOTES							
T NOTES							
W NOTES							
T NOTES							
F NOTES							
S NOTES							
S NOTES							

Week Commencing _____ Feeling ____ / 10

		Breakfast		Lunch		Dinner		Supper
M		BEFORE	AFTER	BEFORE	AFTER	BEFORE	AFTER	BEFORE
	NOTES							
T		BEFORE	AFTER	BEFORE	AFTER	BEFORE	AFTER	BEFORE
	NOTES							
W		BEFORE	AFTER	BEFORE	AFTER	BEFORE	AFTER	BEFORE
	NOTES							
T		BEFORE	AFTER	BEFORE	AFTER	BEFORE	AFTER	BEFORE
	NOTES							
F		BEFORE	AFTER	BEFORE	AFTER	BEFORE	AFTER	BEFORE
	NOTES							
S		BEFORE	AFTER	BEFORE	AFTER	BEFORE	AFTER	BEFORE
	NOTES							
S		BEFORE	AFTER	BEFORE	AFTER	BEFORE	AFTER	BEFORE
	NOTES							

Week Commencing _____   Feeling _____ / 10

	Breakfast		Lunch		Dinner		Supper
	BEFORE	AFTER	BEFORE	AFTER	BEFORE	AFTER	BEFORE
M NOTES							
T NOTES							
W NOTES							
T NOTES							
F NOTES							
S NOTES							
S NOTES							

Week Commencing _____   Feeling _____ / 10

	Breakfast		Lunch		Dinner		Supper
	BEFORE	AFTER	BEFORE	AFTER	BEFORE	AFTER	BEFORE
M							
NOTES							
T	BEFORE	AFTER	BEFORE	AFTER	BEFORE	AFTER	BEFORE
NOTES							
W	BEFORE	AFTER	BEFORE	AFTER	BEFORE	AFTER	BEFORE
NOTES							
T	BEFORE	AFTER	BEFORE	AFTER	BEFORE	AFTER	BEFORE
NOTES							
F	BEFORE	AFTER	BEFORE	AFTER	BEFORE	AFTER	BEFORE
NOTES							
S	BEFORE	AFTER	BEFORE	AFTER	BEFORE	AFTER	BEFORE
NOTES							
S	BEFORE	AFTER	BEFORE	AFTER	BEFORE	AFTER	BEFORE
NOTES							

Week Commencing _____   Feeling _____ / 10

	Breakfast		Lunch		Dinner		Supper
	BEFORE	AFTER	BEFORE	AFTER	BEFORE	AFTER	BEFORE
M NOTES							
T NOTES							
W NOTES							
T NOTES							
F NOTES							
S NOTES							
S NOTES							

Week Commencing _____   Feeling _____ / 10

	Breakfast		Lunch		Dinner		Supper
	BEFORE	AFTER	BEFORE	AFTER	BEFORE	AFTER	BEFORE
M							
NOTES							
T							
NOTES							
W							
NOTES							
T							
NOTES							
F							
NOTES							
S							
NOTES							
S							
NOTES							

Week Commencing _____   Feeling ____ / 10

	Breakfast		Lunch		Dinner		Supper
	BEFORE	AFTER	BEFORE	AFTER	BEFORE	AFTER	BEFORE
M NOTES							
T NOTES							
W NOTES							
T NOTES							
F NOTES							
S NOTES							
S NOTES							

Week Commencing _____   Feeling _____ / 10

	Breakfast		Lunch		Dinner		Supper
	BEFORE	AFTER	BEFORE	AFTER	BEFORE	AFTER	BEFORE
M							
NOTES							
	BEFORE	AFTER	BEFORE	AFTER	BEFORE	AFTER	BEFORE
T							
NOTES							
	BEFORE	AFTER	BEFORE	AFTER	BEFORE	AFTER	BEFORE
W							
NOTES							
	BEFORE	AFTER	BEFORE	AFTER	BEFORE	AFTER	BEFORE
T							
NOTES							
	BEFORE	AFTER	BEFORE	AFTER	BEFORE	AFTER	BEFORE
F							
NOTES							
	BEFORE	AFTER	BEFORE	AFTER	BEFORE	AFTER	BEFORE
S							
NOTES							
	BEFORE	AFTER	BEFORE	AFTER	BEFORE	AFTER	BEFORE
S							
NOTES							

Week Commencing _____   Feeling _____ / 10

	Breakfast		Lunch		Dinner		Supper
	BEFORE	AFTER	BEFORE	AFTER	BEFORE	AFTER	BEFORE
M NOTES							
	BEFORE	AFTER	BEFORE	AFTER	BEFORE	AFTER	BEFORE
T NOTES							
	BEFORE	AFTER	BEFORE	AFTER	BEFORE	AFTER	BEFORE
W NOTES							
	BEFORE	AFTER	BEFORE	AFTER	BEFORE	AFTER	BEFORE
T NOTES							
	BEFORE	AFTER	BEFORE	AFTER	BEFORE	AFTER	BEFORE
F NOTES							
	BEFORE	AFTER	BEFORE	AFTER	BEFORE	AFTER	BEFORE
S NOTES							
	BEFORE	AFTER	BEFORE	AFTER	BEFORE	AFTER	BEFORE
S NOTES							

Week Commencing _____   Feeling _____ / 10

	Breakfast		Lunch		Dinner		Supper
	BEFORE	AFTER	BEFORE	AFTER	BEFORE	AFTER	BEFORE
M NOTES							
T NOTES							
W NOTES							
T NOTES							
F NOTES							
S NOTES							
S NOTES							

Week Commencing _____   Feeling _____ / 10

	Breakfast		Lunch		Dinner		Supper
	BEFORE	AFTER	BEFORE	AFTER	BEFORE	AFTER	BEFORE
M							
NOTES							
	BEFORE	AFTER	BEFORE	AFTER	BEFORE	AFTER	BEFORE
T							
NOTES							
	BEFORE	AFTER	BEFORE	AFTER	BEFORE	AFTER	BEFORE
W							
NOTES							
	BEFORE	AFTER	BEFORE	AFTER	BEFORE	AFTER	BEFORE
T							
NOTES							
	BEFORE	AFTER	BEFORE	AFTER	BEFORE	AFTER	BEFORE
F							
NOTES							
	BEFORE	AFTER	BEFORE	AFTER	BEFORE	AFTER	BEFORE
S							
NOTES							
	BEFORE	AFTER	BEFORE	AFTER	BEFORE	AFTER	BEFORE
S							
NOTES							

Week Commencing _____   Feeling _____ / 10

	Breakfast		Lunch		Dinner		Supper
	BEFORE	AFTER	BEFORE	AFTER	BEFORE	AFTER	BEFORE
M							
NOTES							
	BEFORE	AFTER	BEFORE	AFTER	BEFORE	AFTER	BEFORE
T							
NOTES							
	BEFORE	AFTER	BEFORE	AFTER	BEFORE	AFTER	BEFORE
W							
NOTES							
	BEFORE	AFTER	BEFORE	AFTER	BEFORE	AFTER	BEFORE
T							
NOTES							
	BEFORE	AFTER	BEFORE	AFTER	BEFORE	AFTER	BEFORE
F							
NOTES							
	BEFORE	AFTER	BEFORE	AFTER	BEFORE	AFTER	BEFORE
S							
NOTES							
	BEFORE	AFTER	BEFORE	AFTER	BEFORE	AFTER	BEFORE
S							
NOTES							

Week Commencing _____   Feeling ____ / 10

	Breakfast		Lunch		Dinner		Supper
	BEFORE	AFTER	BEFORE	AFTER	BEFORE	AFTER	BEFORE
M							
NOTES							
T	BEFORE	AFTER	BEFORE	AFTER	BEFORE	AFTER	BEFORE
NOTES							
W	BEFORE	AFTER	BEFORE	AFTER	BEFORE	AFTER	BEFORE
NOTES							
T	BEFORE	AFTER	BEFORE	AFTER	BEFORE	AFTER	BEFORE
NOTES							
F	BEFORE	AFTER	BEFORE	AFTER	BEFORE	AFTER	BEFORE
NOTES							
S	BEFORE	AFTER	BEFORE	AFTER	BEFORE	AFTER	BEFORE
NOTES							
S	BEFORE	AFTER	BEFORE	AFTER	BEFORE	AFTER	BEFORE
NOTES							

Week Commencing _____   Feeling _____ / 10

	Breakfast		Lunch		Dinner		Supper
	BEFORE	AFTER	BEFORE	AFTER	BEFORE	AFTER	BEFORE
M							
NOTES							
T	BEFORE	AFTER	BEFORE	AFTER	BEFORE	AFTER	BEFORE
NOTES							
W	BEFORE	AFTER	BEFORE	AFTER	BEFORE	AFTER	BEFORE
NOTES							
T	BEFORE	AFTER	BEFORE	AFTER	BEFORE	AFTER	BEFORE
NOTES							
F	BEFORE	AFTER	BEFORE	AFTER	BEFORE	AFTER	BEFORE
NOTES							
S	BEFORE	AFTER	BEFORE	AFTER	BEFORE	AFTER	BEFORE
NOTES							
S	BEFORE	AFTER	BEFORE	AFTER	BEFORE	AFTER	BEFORE
NOTES							

Week Commencing _____   Feeling _____ / 10

	Breakfast		Lunch		Dinner		Supper
	BEFORE	AFTER	BEFORE	AFTER	BEFORE	AFTER	BEFORE
M							
NOTES							
T							
NOTES							
W							
NOTES							
T							
NOTES							
F							
NOTES							
S							
NOTES							
S							
NOTES							

Week Commencing _____ Feeling _____ / 10

	Breakfast		Lunch		Dinner		Supper
	BEFORE	AFTER	BEFORE	AFTER	BEFORE	AFTER	BEFORE
M							
NOTES							
T	BEFORE	AFTER	BEFORE	AFTER	BEFORE	AFTER	BEFORE
NOTES							
W	BEFORE	AFTER	BEFORE	AFTER	BEFORE	AFTER	BEFORE
NOTES							
T	BEFORE	AFTER	BEFORE	AFTER	BEFORE	AFTER	BEFORE
NOTES							
F	BEFORE	AFTER	BEFORE	AFTER	BEFORE	AFTER	BEFORE
NOTES							
S	BEFORE	AFTER	BEFORE	AFTER	BEFORE	AFTER	BEFORE
NOTES							
S	BEFORE	AFTER	BEFORE	AFTER	BEFORE	AFTER	BEFORE
NOTES							

Week Commencing _____   Feeling ____ / 10

	Breakfast		Lunch		Dinner		Supper
	BEFORE	AFTER	BEFORE	AFTER	BEFORE	AFTER	BEFORE
M							
NOTES							
	BEFORE	AFTER	BEFORE	AFTER	BEFORE	AFTER	BEFORE
T							
NOTES							
	BEFORE	AFTER	BEFORE	AFTER	BEFORE	AFTER	BEFORE
W							
NOTES							
	BEFORE	AFTER	BEFORE	AFTER	BEFORE	AFTER	BEFORE
T							
NOTES							
	BEFORE	AFTER	BEFORE	AFTER	BEFORE	AFTER	BEFORE
F							
NOTES							
	BEFORE	AFTER	BEFORE	AFTER	BEFORE	AFTER	BEFORE
S							
NOTES							
	BEFORE	AFTER	BEFORE	AFTER	BEFORE	AFTER	BEFORE
S							
NOTES							

Week Commencing _____   Feeling ____ / 10

	Breakfast		Lunch		Dinner		Supper
	BEFORE	AFTER	BEFORE	AFTER	BEFORE	AFTER	BEFORE
M							
NOTES							
T	BEFORE	AFTER	BEFORE	AFTER	BEFORE	AFTER	BEFORE
NOTES							
W	BEFORE	AFTER	BEFORE	AFTER	BEFORE	AFTER	BEFORE
NOTES							
T	BEFORE	AFTER	BEFORE	AFTER	BEFORE	AFTER	BEFORE
NOTES							
F	BEFORE	AFTER	BEFORE	AFTER	BEFORE	AFTER	BEFORE
NOTES							
S	BEFORE	AFTER	BEFORE	AFTER	BEFORE	AFTER	BEFORE
NOTES							
S	BEFORE	AFTER	BEFORE	AFTER	BEFORE	AFTER	BEFORE
NOTES							

Week Commencing _____   Feeling _____ / 10

	Breakfast		Lunch		Dinner		Supper
	BEFORE	AFTER	BEFORE	AFTER	BEFORE	AFTER	BEFORE
M							
NOTES							
T	BEFORE	AFTER	BEFORE	AFTER	BEFORE	AFTER	BEFORE
NOTES							
W	BEFORE	AFTER	BEFORE	AFTER	BEFORE	AFTER	BEFORE
NOTES							
T	BEFORE	AFTER	BEFORE	AFTER	BEFORE	AFTER	BEFORE
NOTES							
F	BEFORE	AFTER	BEFORE	AFTER	BEFORE	AFTER	BEFORE
NOTES							
S	BEFORE	AFTER	BEFORE	AFTER	BEFORE	AFTER	BEFORE
NOTES							
S	BEFORE	AFTER	BEFORE	AFTER	BEFORE	AFTER	BEFORE
NOTES							

Week Commencing _____   Feeling _____ / 10

	Breakfast		Lunch		Dinner		Supper
	BEFORE	AFTER	BEFORE	AFTER	BEFORE	AFTER	BEFORE
M							
NOTES							
T	BEFORE	AFTER	BEFORE	AFTER	BEFORE	AFTER	BEFORE
NOTES							
W	BEFORE	AFTER	BEFORE	AFTER	BEFORE	AFTER	BEFORE
NOTES							
T	BEFORE	AFTER	BEFORE	AFTER	BEFORE	AFTER	BEFORE
NOTES							
F	BEFORE	AFTER	BEFORE	AFTER	BEFORE	AFTER	BEFORE
NOTES							
S	BEFORE	AFTER	BEFORE	AFTER	BEFORE	AFTER	BEFORE
NOTES							
S	BEFORE	AFTER	BEFORE	AFTER	BEFORE	AFTER	BEFORE
NOTES							

Week Commencing _____   Feeling ____ / 10

	Breakfast		Lunch		Dinner		Supper
	BEFORE	AFTER	BEFORE	AFTER	BEFORE	AFTER	BEFORE
M							
NOTES							
T	BEFORE	AFTER	BEFORE	AFTER	BEFORE	AFTER	BEFORE
NOTES							
W	BEFORE	AFTER	BEFORE	AFTER	BEFORE	AFTER	BEFORE
NOTES							
T	BEFORE	AFTER	BEFORE	AFTER	BEFORE	AFTER	BEFORE
NOTES							
F	BEFORE	AFTER	BEFORE	AFTER	BEFORE	AFTER	BEFORE
NOTES							
S	BEFORE	AFTER	BEFORE	AFTER	BEFORE	AFTER	BEFORE
NOTES							
S	BEFORE	AFTER	BEFORE	AFTER	BEFORE	AFTER	BEFORE
NOTES							

Week Commencing _____   Feeling ____ / 10

		Breakfast		Lunch		Dinner		Supper
		BEFORE	AFTER	BEFORE	AFTER	BEFORE	AFTER	BEFORE
M								
NOTES								
		BEFORE	AFTER	BEFORE	AFTER	BEFORE	AFTER	BEFORE
T								
NOTES								
		BEFORE	AFTER	BEFORE	AFTER	BEFORE	AFTER	BEFORE
W								
NOTES								
		BEFORE	AFTER	BEFORE	AFTER	BEFORE	AFTER	BEFORE
T								
NOTES								
		BEFORE	AFTER	BEFORE	AFTER	BEFORE	AFTER	BEFORE
F								
NOTES								
		BEFORE	AFTER	BEFORE	AFTER	BEFORE	AFTER	BEFORE
S								
NOTES								
		BEFORE	AFTER	BEFORE	AFTER	BEFORE	AFTER	BEFORE
S								
NOTES								

Week Commencing _____ Feeling ____ / 10

	Breakfast		Lunch		Dinner		Supper
	BEFORE	AFTER	BEFORE	AFTER	BEFORE	AFTER	BEFORE
M							
NOTES							
T	BEFORE	AFTER	BEFORE	AFTER	BEFORE	AFTER	BEFORE
NOTES							
W	BEFORE	AFTER	BEFORE	AFTER	BEFORE	AFTER	BEFORE
NOTES							
T	BEFORE	AFTER	BEFORE	AFTER	BEFORE	AFTER	BEFORE
NOTES							
F	BEFORE	AFTER	BEFORE	AFTER	BEFORE	AFTER	BEFORE
NOTES							
S	BEFORE	AFTER	BEFORE	AFTER	BEFORE	AFTER	BEFORE
NOTES							
S	BEFORE	AFTER	BEFORE	AFTER	BEFORE	AFTER	BEFORE
NOTES							

Week Commencing _____   Feeling _____ / 10

	Breakfast		Lunch		Dinner		Supper
	BEFORE	AFTER	BEFORE	AFTER	BEFORE	AFTER	BEFORE
M							
NOTES							
	BEFORE	AFTER	BEFORE	AFTER	BEFORE	AFTER	BEFORE
T							
NOTES							
	BEFORE	AFTER	BEFORE	AFTER	BEFORE	AFTER	BEFORE
W							
NOTES							
	BEFORE	AFTER	BEFORE	AFTER	BEFORE	AFTER	BEFORE
T							
NOTES							
	BEFORE	AFTER	BEFORE	AFTER	BEFORE	AFTER	BEFORE
F							
NOTES							
	BEFORE	AFTER	BEFORE	AFTER	BEFORE	AFTER	BEFORE
S							
NOTES							
	BEFORE	AFTER	BEFORE	AFTER	BEFORE	AFTER	BEFORE
S							
NOTES							

Week Commencing _____   Feeling ____ / 10

	Breakfast		Lunch		Dinner		Supper
	BEFORE	AFTER	BEFORE	AFTER	BEFORE	AFTER	BEFORE
M NOTES							
T NOTES							
W NOTES							
T NOTES							
F NOTES							
S NOTES							
S NOTES							

Week Commencing _____   Feeling ____ / 10

	Breakfast		Lunch		Dinner		Supper
	BEFORE	AFTER	BEFORE	AFTER	BEFORE	AFTER	BEFORE
M NOTES							
T NOTES							
W NOTES							
T NOTES							
F NOTES							
S NOTES							
S NOTES							

Week Commencing _____   Feeling _____ / 10

	Breakfast		Lunch		Dinner		Supper
	BEFORE	AFTER	BEFORE	AFTER	BEFORE	AFTER	BEFORE
M							
NOTES							
	BEFORE	AFTER	BEFORE	AFTER	BEFORE	AFTER	BEFORE
T							
NOTES							
	BEFORE	AFTER	BEFORE	AFTER	BEFORE	AFTER	BEFORE
W							
NOTES							
	BEFORE	AFTER	BEFORE	AFTER	BEFORE	AFTER	BEFORE
T							
NOTES							
	BEFORE	AFTER	BEFORE	AFTER	BEFORE	AFTER	BEFORE
F							
NOTES							
	BEFORE	AFTER	BEFORE	AFTER	BEFORE	AFTER	BEFORE
S							
NOTES							
	BEFORE	AFTER	BEFORE	AFTER	BEFORE	AFTER	BEFORE
S							
NOTES							

Week Commencing _____ Feeling _____ / 10

	Breakfast		Lunch		Dinner		Supper
	BEFORE	AFTER	BEFORE	AFTER	BEFORE	AFTER	BEFORE
M NOTES							
T NOTES							
W NOTES							
T NOTES							
F NOTES							
S NOTES							
S NOTES							

Week Commencing _____   Feeling _____ / 10

	Breakfast		Lunch		Dinner		Supper
	BEFORE	AFTER	BEFORE	AFTER	BEFORE	AFTER	BEFORE
M							
NOTES							
T	BEFORE	AFTER	BEFORE	AFTER	BEFORE	AFTER	BEFORE
NOTES							
W	BEFORE	AFTER	BEFORE	AFTER	BEFORE	AFTER	BEFORE
NOTES							
T	BEFORE	AFTER	BEFORE	AFTER	BEFORE	AFTER	BEFORE
NOTES							
F	BEFORE	AFTER	BEFORE	AFTER	BEFORE	AFTER	BEFORE
NOTES							
S	BEFORE	AFTER	BEFORE	AFTER	BEFORE	AFTER	BEFORE
NOTES							
S	BEFORE	AFTER	BEFORE	AFTER	BEFORE	AFTER	BEFORE
NOTES							

Week Commencing _____   Feeling _____ / 10

	Breakfast		Lunch		Dinner		Supper
	BEFORE	AFTER	BEFORE	AFTER	BEFORE	AFTER	BEFORE
M							
NOTES							
	BEFORE	AFTER	BEFORE	AFTER	BEFORE	AFTER	BEFORE
T							
NOTES							
	BEFORE	AFTER	BEFORE	AFTER	BEFORE	AFTER	BEFORE
W							
NOTES							
	BEFORE	AFTER	BEFORE	AFTER	BEFORE	AFTER	BEFORE
T							
NOTES							
	BEFORE	AFTER	BEFORE	AFTER	BEFORE	AFTER	BEFORE
F							
NOTES							
	BEFORE	AFTER	BEFORE	AFTER	BEFORE	AFTER	BEFORE
S							
NOTES							
	BEFORE	AFTER	BEFORE	AFTER	BEFORE	AFTER	BEFORE
S							
NOTES							

Week Commencing _____   Feeling ____ / 10

	Breakfast		Lunch		Dinner		Supper
	BEFORE	AFTER	BEFORE	AFTER	BEFORE	AFTER	BEFORE
M NOTES							
T NOTES							
W NOTES							
T NOTES							
F NOTES							
S NOTES							
S NOTES							

Week Commencing _____   Feeling _____ / 10

	Breakfast		Lunch		Dinner		Supper
M	BEFORE	AFTER	BEFORE	AFTER	BEFORE	AFTER	BEFORE
NOTES							
T	BEFORE	AFTER	BEFORE	AFTER	BEFORE	AFTER	BEFORE
NOTES							
W	BEFORE	AFTER	BEFORE	AFTER	BEFORE	AFTER	BEFORE
NOTES							
T	BEFORE	AFTER	BEFORE	AFTER	BEFORE	AFTER	BEFORE
NOTES							
F	BEFORE	AFTER	BEFORE	AFTER	BEFORE	AFTER	BEFORE
NOTES							
S	BEFORE	AFTER	BEFORE	AFTER	BEFORE	AFTER	BEFORE
NOTES							
S	BEFORE	AFTER	BEFORE	AFTER	BEFORE	AFTER	BEFORE
NOTES							

Week Commencing _____   Feeling ____ / 10

	Breakfast		Lunch		Dinner		Supper
	BEFORE	AFTER	BEFORE	AFTER	BEFORE	AFTER	BEFORE
M							
NOTES							
T							
NOTES							
W							
NOTES							
T							
NOTES							
F							
NOTES							
S							
NOTES							
S							
NOTES							

Week Commencing _____   Feeling _____ / 10

	Breakfast		Lunch		Dinner		Supper
	BEFORE	AFTER	BEFORE	AFTER	BEFORE	AFTER	BEFORE
M							
NOTES							
	BEFORE	AFTER	BEFORE	AFTER	BEFORE	AFTER	BEFORE
T							
NOTES							
	BEFORE	AFTER	BEFORE	AFTER	BEFORE	AFTER	BEFORE
W							
NOTES							
	BEFORE	AFTER	BEFORE	AFTER	BEFORE	AFTER	BEFORE
T							
NOTES							
	BEFORE	AFTER	BEFORE	AFTER	BEFORE	AFTER	BEFORE
F							
NOTES							
	BEFORE	AFTER	BEFORE	AFTER	BEFORE	AFTER	BEFORE
S							
NOTES							
	BEFORE	AFTER	BEFORE	AFTER	BEFORE	AFTER	BEFORE
S							
NOTES							

Week Commencing _____   Feeling ____ / 10

	Breakfast		Lunch		Dinner		Supper
	BEFORE	AFTER	BEFORE	AFTER	BEFORE	AFTER	BEFORE
M							
NOTES							
	BEFORE	AFTER	BEFORE	AFTER	BEFORE	AFTER	BEFORE
T							
NOTES							
	BEFORE	AFTER	BEFORE	AFTER	BEFORE	AFTER	BEFORE
W							
NOTES							
	BEFORE	AFTER	BEFORE	AFTER	BEFORE	AFTER	BEFORE
T							
NOTES							
	BEFORE	AFTER	BEFORE	AFTER	BEFORE	AFTER	BEFORE
F							
NOTES							
	BEFORE	AFTER	BEFORE	AFTER	BEFORE	AFTER	BEFORE
S							
NOTES							
	BEFORE	AFTER	BEFORE	AFTER	BEFORE	AFTER	BEFORE
S							
NOTES							

Week Commencing _____   Feeling ____ / 10

	Breakfast		Lunch		Dinner		Supper
	BEFORE	AFTER	BEFORE	AFTER	BEFORE	AFTER	BEFORE
M							
NOTES							
T							
NOTES							
W							
NOTES							
T							
NOTES							
F							
NOTES							
S							
NOTES							
S							
NOTES							

Week Commencing _____   Feeling _____ / 10

	Breakfast		Lunch		Dinner		Supper
	BEFORE	AFTER	BEFORE	AFTER	BEFORE	AFTER	BEFORE
M NOTES							
T NOTES							
W NOTES							
T NOTES							
F NOTES							
S NOTES							
S NOTES							

Week Commencing _____   Feeling _____ / 10

	Breakfast		Lunch		Dinner		Supper
	BEFORE	AFTER	BEFORE	AFTER	BEFORE	AFTER	BEFORE
M NOTES							
T NOTES							
W NOTES							
T NOTES							
F NOTES							
S NOTES							
S NOTES							

Week Commencing _____   Feeling _____ / 10

	Breakfast		Lunch		Dinner		Supper
	BEFORE	AFTER	BEFORE	AFTER	BEFORE	AFTER	BEFORE
M							
NOTES							
	BEFORE	AFTER	BEFORE	AFTER	BEFORE	AFTER	BEFORE
T							
NOTES							
	BEFORE	AFTER	BEFORE	AFTER	BEFORE	AFTER	BEFORE
W							
NOTES							
	BEFORE	AFTER	BEFORE	AFTER	BEFORE	AFTER	BEFORE
T							
NOTES							
	BEFORE	AFTER	BEFORE	AFTER	BEFORE	AFTER	BEFORE
F							
NOTES							
	BEFORE	AFTER	BEFORE	AFTER	BEFORE	AFTER	BEFORE
S							
NOTES							
	BEFORE	AFTER	BEFORE	AFTER	BEFORE	AFTER	BEFORE
S							
NOTES							

Week Commencing _____   Feeling _____ / 10

	Breakfast		Lunch		Dinner		Supper
	BEFORE	AFTER	BEFORE	AFTER	BEFORE	AFTER	BEFORE
M							
NOTES							
	BEFORE	AFTER	BEFORE	AFTER	BEFORE	AFTER	BEFORE
T							
NOTES							
	BEFORE	AFTER	BEFORE	AFTER	BEFORE	AFTER	BEFORE
W							
NOTES							
	BEFORE	AFTER	BEFORE	AFTER	BEFORE	AFTER	BEFORE
T							
NOTES							
	BEFORE	AFTER	BEFORE	AFTER	BEFORE	AFTER	BEFORE
F							
NOTES							
	BEFORE	AFTER	BEFORE	AFTER	BEFORE	AFTER	BEFORE
S							
NOTES							
	BEFORE	AFTER	BEFORE	AFTER	BEFORE	AFTER	BEFORE
S							
NOTES							

Week Commencing _____ Feeling ___ / 10

	Breakfast		Lunch		Dinner		Supper
	BEFORE	AFTER	BEFORE	AFTER	BEFORE	AFTER	BEFORE
M							
NOTES							
	BEFORE	AFTER	BEFORE	AFTER	BEFORE	AFTER	BEFORE
T							
NOTES							
	BEFORE	AFTER	BEFORE	AFTER	BEFORE	AFTER	BEFORE
W							
NOTES							
	BEFORE	AFTER	BEFORE	AFTER	BEFORE	AFTER	BEFORE
T							
NOTES							
	BEFORE	AFTER	BEFORE	AFTER	BEFORE	AFTER	BEFORE
F							
NOTES							
	BEFORE	AFTER	BEFORE	AFTER	BEFORE	AFTER	BEFORE
S							
NOTES							
	BEFORE	AFTER	BEFORE	AFTER	BEFORE	AFTER	BEFORE
S							
NOTES							

Week Commencing _____   Feeling _____ / 10

	Breakfast		Lunch		Dinner		Supper
	BEFORE	AFTER	BEFORE	AFTER	BEFORE	AFTER	BEFORE
M							
NOTES							
	BEFORE	AFTER	BEFORE	AFTER	BEFORE	AFTER	BEFORE
T							
NOTES							
	BEFORE	AFTER	BEFORE	AFTER	BEFORE	AFTER	BEFORE
W							
NOTES							
	BEFORE	AFTER	BEFORE	AFTER	BEFORE	AFTER	BEFORE
T							
NOTES							
	BEFORE	AFTER	BEFORE	AFTER	BEFORE	AFTER	BEFORE
F							
NOTES							
	BEFORE	AFTER	BEFORE	AFTER	BEFORE	AFTER	BEFORE
S							
NOTES							
	BEFORE	AFTER	BEFORE	AFTER	BEFORE	AFTER	BEFORE
S							
NOTES							

Week Commencing _____   Feeling _____ / 10

	Breakfast		Lunch		Dinner		Supper
	BEFORE	AFTER	BEFORE	AFTER	BEFORE	AFTER	BEFORE
M NOTES							
T NOTES							
W NOTES							
T NOTES							
F NOTES							
S NOTES							
S NOTES							

Week Commencing _____   Feeling _____ / 10

		Breakfast		Lunch		Dinner		Supper
		BEFORE	AFTER	BEFORE	AFTER	BEFORE	AFTER	BEFORE
M								
NOTES								
		BEFORE	AFTER	BEFORE	AFTER	BEFORE	AFTER	BEFORE
T								
NOTES								
		BEFORE	AFTER	BEFORE	AFTER	BEFORE	AFTER	BEFORE
W								
NOTES								
		BEFORE	AFTER	BEFORE	AFTER	BEFORE	AFTER	BEFORE
T								
NOTES								
		BEFORE	AFTER	BEFORE	AFTER	BEFORE	AFTER	BEFORE
F								
NOTES								
		BEFORE	AFTER	BEFORE	AFTER	BEFORE	AFTER	BEFORE
S								
NOTES								
		BEFORE	AFTER	BEFORE	AFTER	BEFORE	AFTER	BEFORE
S								
NOTES								

Week Commencing _____   Feeling _____ / 10

	Breakfast		Lunch		Dinner		Supper
	BEFORE	AFTER	BEFORE	AFTER	BEFORE	AFTER	BEFORE
M NOTES							
T NOTES	BEFORE	AFTER	BEFORE	AFTER	BEFORE	AFTER	BEFORE
W NOTES	BEFORE	AFTER	BEFORE	AFTER	BEFORE	AFTER	BEFORE
T NOTES	BEFORE	AFTER	BEFORE	AFTER	BEFORE	AFTER	BEFORE
F NOTES	BEFORE	AFTER	BEFORE	AFTER	BEFORE	AFTER	BEFORE
S NOTES	BEFORE	AFTER	BEFORE	AFTER	BEFORE	AFTER	BEFORE
S NOTES	BEFORE	AFTER	BEFORE	AFTER	BEFORE	AFTER	BEFORE

Week Commencing _____   Feeling _____ / 10

	Breakfast		Lunch		Dinner		Supper
	BEFORE	AFTER	BEFORE	AFTER	BEFORE	AFTER	BEFORE
M NOTES							
T NOTES							
W NOTES							
T NOTES							
F NOTES							
S NOTES							
S NOTES							

Week Commencing _____   Feeling _____ / 10

	Breakfast		Lunch		Dinner		Supper
	BEFORE	AFTER	BEFORE	AFTER	BEFORE	AFTER	BEFORE
M							
NOTES							
T							
NOTES							
W							
NOTES							
T							
NOTES							
F							
NOTES							
S							
NOTES							
S							
NOTES							

Manufactured by Amazon.ca
Bolton, ON